HOW'S YOUR
BACK?

HOW'S YOUR BACK?

VIRGILIO V. FLORES

To order additional copies of this book, contact:
Xlibris Corporation
1-888-795-4274
www.Xlibris.com
Orders@Xlibris.com
104480

Contents

Introduction

Three decades or so ago, I unintentionally joined the legion of common low back pain sufferers all over the world. My common low back pain started innocuously enough, a little pain here, a little pain there. The pain gradually increased to the point that I could not ignore it any longer. The one thing that I was sure of was that I did not want to have surgery on my back. Any spine surgery requiring general anesthesia would hurt a lot for weeks to months. I was afraid of pain after surgery. Besides, I knew several patients who had back surgery and still had recurrence of back pain anyways. A few unfortunate victims had pain that did not go away at all even after surgery. These unfortunate victims became incapacitated and disabled by the pain. Additionally, I did not want to be addicted to painkillers. A dilemma presented itself. What can I do to relieve my low back pain without painkillers or surgery? Fortunately for me, I stumbled onto a life-changing discovery.

By the way, how does my book title grab you? To answer my own question, I would say, "My back is fine, thank you very much! How about yours?" My back is fine and will be fine for a long time to come and shall last my entire lifetime thankfully, due to the life-changing discovery I just mentioned that consisted of combining gravity traction (inversion) and exercises. I discovered this method over twenty-five years ago "in a flash of genius," one might say. I benefited tremendously from this method. I kept it a closely guarded secret for many years until now.

I have noticed for many years that people buy gravity inversion tables (machines/ equipments) with the hope of getting rid of their common low back pain. The keyword here is *hope*. You can hope all you want, but if you do not do something and combine *hope* with *action*, you will never get rid of your common low back pain. You cannot just get on the inversion table, get inverted, and just hang there and *hope* your common low back pain will disappear instantly or eventually. In addition, you cannot let a little pain, nausea, dizziness, headache, and/ or feeling terribly ill discourage you from ever getting on the inversion table again and again to achieve your goal of getting rid of your common low back pain. However, I have no verifiable scientific data to explain why my method works so well. It just works very well for me. It is my hope that after you try my method your common back pain will be a thing of the past like mine. My method is like acupuncture: it works with perfection without any definitive scientific explanation.

It is not my intention to sell you gadgets, widgets, lotions, potions, snake oil, machines, or fancy equipments to treat your common low back pain. You buy, borrow, or rent those on your own. What I want to do for you is to share with you my knowledge. This will make it possible for you to get rid of your own common low back pain once it appears and subsequently recurs again. One thing is guaranteed: that is, once you have common low back pain, it will recur again. But not to worry. Another sure thing I know is that once you have recurrence of low back pain, it is comforting to know that you can get rid of it in one session lasting just ninety seconds if it is a minor pain. And up to three days if it is a major pain that would otherwise require surgery to get rid of. But of course, you are free to choose surgery for acute severe low back pain.

(And more) just means I am giving you, my reader, a few more suggestions of what works for me and/or others outside of common low back pain.

Chapter 1

THE EARLY YEARS

I knew in my mid-twenties (circa 1974) that I was going to suffer from common low back pain, also called chronic back pain syndrome in medical terms, later in life. I was a medical student at the University of Hawaii Medical School. A clinical professor (an orthopedic surgeon) in my physical examination class at Tripler Army Medical Center, Honolulu, Hawaii, predicted in class that I would have common low back pain when I grew older because my right leg was shorter than my left leg. I was very skeptical of this prediction. It was not until I was in my mid-thirties while serving as a US Navy anesthesiologist at Long Beach Naval Regional Medical Center, Long Beach, California, that I slowly but progressively began developing increasingly severe common low back pain. I could not help but remember what that professor had said. His prediction was coming true with a vengeance.

"What do I do now?" I asked myself. I did not want to be addicted to painkiller medications. More importantly, I did not want surgery. The thought of having back surgery terrified me. I vowed to myself: no painkillers and no surgery.

Being a medical doctor gave me an edge. I approached common low back pain as a mechanical problem with physiological consequences. Armed with that knowledge, I vowed to do something. Anything. But what? I discovered a method, simple yet so effective. It amazed me that to this day only a few fortunate souls have serendipitously discovered for themselves my method. My method combined SPINE TRACTION using gravity (also called gravity inversion) with EXERCISES. Very easily done and very effective. I obtained complete relief from minor to moderate low back pain after a single exercise session lasting only ninety seconds or fewer. I achieved complete relief from very severe common low back pain in only three days, each session lasting only ninety seconds or fewer and only once each day. Very amazing, indeed, since I did not use any medications at all.

I fortunately found out that the EASIEST, CHEAPEST, and FASTEST way to do spine traction was by gravity inversion—a method I came across in the 1970s. Simply put: HANG UPSIDE DOWN. There were machines for gravity inversion sold in the open market at that time.

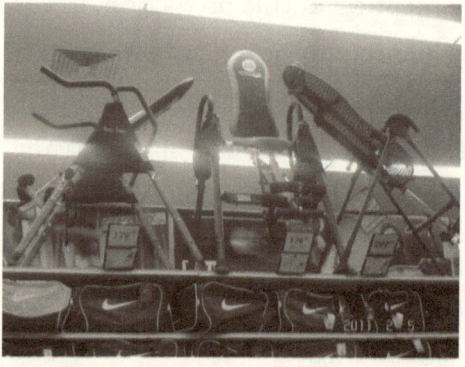

I bought a used gravity inversion equipment that turned out to be one of my best investments of all time.

Chapter 2

SHARING THE GOOD NEWS

Several years had passed since my discovery of the method (combination of gravity inversion and exercise) to obtain complete relief from minor to severe common low back pain. I did not have to worry about recurrent low back pain anymore. With my method, I always achieved complete common low back pain relief. Since my discovery, I always walked pain free, except when I had recurrences, which I dispatched very quickly and completely with my method. I kept the secret within my family for many years. My daughter used to ride horses. She developed common low back pain. She treated her common low back pain successfully with my method. In the last few years, I felt compelled to share my knowledge to a few select friends, namely, Dr. Glenn McFerren, Dr. Raymond Untalan, Felix Abaya Jr., Shawn Morrow, Armando Dominguez, Jerry Suriff (my next-door neighbor), and Nelson Torres, LVN. I wanted to share a good thing. I was also curious to find out for myself if my method worked for others as well. My few select friends are all healthy, gainfully employed, nonsmoking, social drinking, hardworking individuals who just happened to have common low back pain and did not want to have back surgery or forever take pain medications. Incidentally, one of them also had started having bowel and bladder control problems. They all reported back to me that my method beautifully worked for them. I have no explanation why my method works. All I know is that it works like a charm. But do not take my word for it. You have to try my method and find out for yourself if it will work for you too. I must mention also that I had treated my minor neck pains with my method. I achieved complete neck pain relief after one or more exercise sessions lasting up to ninety seconds per session.

Chapter 3

THE GRAVITY INVERSION MACHINE

Several different brands and models of gravity inversion machines can be bought in the open market and on the Internet nowadays. Here in San Angelo, Texas, several models of gravity inversion machines are available at retail stores such as Academy and Big 5.

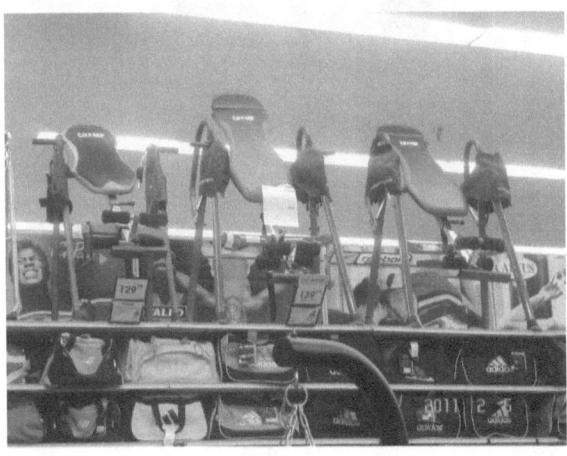

Sam's Club used to sell gravity inversion machines, but not anymore. If you are lucky, you can probably buy one at a garage sale or from a close friend.

I was lucky to buy a used gravity inversion machine back in 1982. It was made of chromed metal with a thick canvas sheet secured to the bed frame by small-diameter nylon ropes. That thing was indestructible. I think it would last forever. My daughter has it now. She still uses it when her low back pain relapses. It came with a special pair of gravity inversion boots made of metal frame and foam insert. More recent gravity inversion boots are made of hard plastic and soft foam, which are very comfortable to wear. A word of caution: the hard plastic boots may break after a few years. The more recent gravity inversion machines do not need special boots anymore.

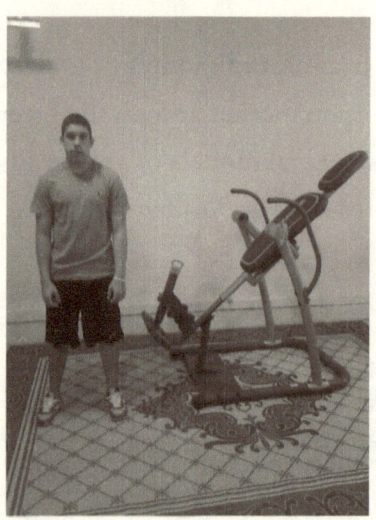

These machines use bars and clamplike contraptions that trap the feet.

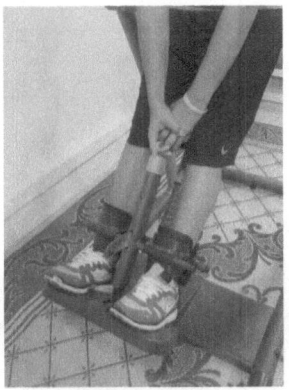

The person using the machine can hang upside down without the need to use special boots. I advise anyone using one of these newer machines to be very careful because your feet can slip off. You can fall headfirst and break your neck and become a quadriplegic. It had happened to some unfortunate individual. Beware. And I strongly recommend using ordinary shoes or boots when you hang upside down with these newer gravity inversion machines.

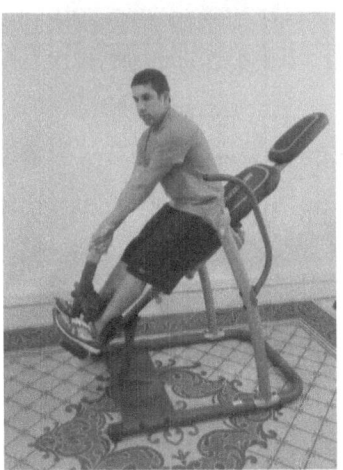

I believe shoes or, more preferably, boots will aid the machine to trap your feet better so you don't fall headfirst. An alternative would be to tie your feet to the bars with Velcro straps. I have not tried this technique. It is up to you to try this one at your own risk.

Chapter 4

THE DISCLAIMER

Before I proceed, I have to give you, my reader, my disclaimer. I wrote this book with the hope that by sharing with you my experiences with my own common low back pain and neck pain, you can learn from them and achieve relief from your own common low back pain and neck pain. I have to strongly warn you that my method will not work for everyone. If you cannot get into the proper position or have no desire to do so, you have no *hope* of achieving common low back pain or neck pain relief. There are many conditions that will prevent you from being upside down, hanging by your ankles. For example, extreme obesity, uncontrolled high blood pressure, acute or chronic heart failure, more advanced cancer, acute or non-healed spine fracture, acute whiplash injury, osteoporosis, severe scoliosis, kyphosis, severe arthritis, brain aneurysm, vertebral body bone spurs, second and third trimester of pregnancy, fear of hanging upside down, to name a few. If you want to try my method, *you do it entirely at your own risk.* In addition, my method requires that you invest in a little pain to eliminate a much larger pain. It can be very painful to get into the proper position on the gravity inversion equipment during an acute attack of severe common low back pain. I strongly recommend you consult your own physician if you can hang upside down. Follow his advice. If your physician gives you the go-ahead, have another person help you get into the proper position. Having said that and if there are no contraindications for you to hang upside down, the rewards are great—no back and/or neck pain.

Chapter 5

THE METHOD

I started applying my method to myself using a special gravity inversion pair of boots, made of metal frame and foam inserts. My family used to live in a small house at Conquista Avenue, Long Beach, California. That house had a narrow doorway and hallway leading to the two bedrooms. I installed a chin-up bar up high between the opposing sides (doorjamb) of the doorway. The boots had special hooks in front that attached to the chin-up bar that enabled me to hang upside down. I placed a big rope midway on the bar with knots at six-inch intervals. I used this rope to pull myself up from the inverted position and off the chin-up bar after my exercises. I graduated to using a gravity inversion machine after I purchased a used one. My method consists of a series of exercises that I perform while hanging upside down by my ankles. When I started doing my gravity inversion exercises, I could hang upside down for only two minutes. It hurt like crazy in my ankles after that. Initially, I thought that maybe it would not do my back any good if I could assume the upside down position for only two minutes, sometimes less. But fortunately for me, I was wrong. It took only up to ninety seconds to do all my exercises. The results were phenomenal. I achieved complete common low back pain relief after a week of daily ninety-second exercise sessions.

Initially, I did not have names for my exercises. I just did several series of movements that worked perfectly well for me. I did at most ten repetitions for each set of exercises, sometimes less. Eventually I found out that ten repetitions were most effective and beneficial for me. You can do more repetitions if you like, but that is entirely up to you. The minor low back pain and/or neck pain relief I achieved with gravity inversion exercises was immediate and longer lasting compared to taking any muscle relaxant or pain medication available in the market today.

In order to perform my exercises properly, you must assume the proper position on the gravity inversion machine. You must have somebody else help you get into the proper position. After you gain experience getting into position on the gravity inversion machine, you may be able to get on it by yourself. I will not recommend that you do it alone, but I have done it. The proper position is a must in order to achieve the most benefit from hanging upside down. You must be suspended by your ankles at ninety degrees from horizontal. However, you can still obtain limited relief even if you hang head down less than ninety degrees. It just takes a bit longer to achieve relief. The closer your body position is to ninety degrees from horizontal, the more relief you will achieve in shorter period of time. Unfortunately, you will also hurt more, especially if you are experiencing severe acute common low back pain. During an acute attack of severe low back pain, hanging upside down at ninety degrees is pure torture, so a position less than ninety degrees might just be the break that you need. The relief from severe acute low back pain is minimal with less than ninety degrees of body inclination, but you will still make some progress. And it will take more than a few days to achieve complete relief. You can progress toward hanging fully by your ankles at ninety degrees in three days. While you are hanging upside down, you have to do something with your hands to help you apply more traction to your back and neck. Your hands and arms can easily weigh more than a couple of pounds especially if you are a large individual. What I did was to hook my thumbs on opposing sides of my jaw, spread the tips of my remaining fingers on each side of my skull behind my ears in a comfortable position, and let my arms hang comfortably to either side. You have to find for yourself by experimentation this comfortable position.

But before we begin with these exercises, I feel I must share with you one more little secret. After I do my exercises, I always get dizzy, woozy, nauseated, and disoriented when I assume the upright position. I also feel like my head is going to explode. And my eyes "bug out." These sensations are very unpleasant. I am afraid the unpleasant sensations will discourage even the most stalwart individual from doing gravity traction with exercises. I tried several maneuvers to get rid of these unpleasant sensations. Through trial and error, I found the most effective and quickest way to get rid of the dizziness and other unpleasant sensations after hanging upside down without using medications. It worked for me all the time. I hope this will work for you too. This is what I do. After I am done with my gravity inversion exercises, I stand up with my hands directly in front of me. I form fists with my fingers. I make like a shadow boxer and strike blow after alternating blow to an imaginary foe in front of me, arms to full extension with each alternating fist strike. I do this series of alternating fist strikes as hard and as fast as I can until I am out of breath and/or I am so tired that I cannot do any more repetitions. I make the blows so hard that my whole body shakes. Then I stop. That's it!

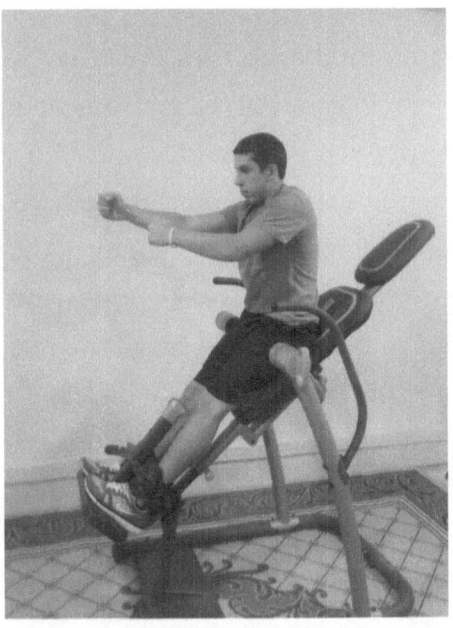

After I had done this, I noticed that my dizziness, nausea, and all other unpleasant sensations were all gone. I could not find faster relief any other way. And it worked for me every time.

My gravity inversion method consists of only five sets of exercises of ten repetitions each. For simplicity's sake, I hereby give each set of exercises a name.

Exercise I

THE TO AND FRO

It is time to begin with the exercises. If you have severe common low back pain, I strongly recommend you get somebody's help to get into position on the gravity inversion machine. Even if your common low back pain is only minor, I still recommend you have another person to help you get into position. You can choose any of the following five sets of exercises to begin your journey to your achievement of common low back pain relief, but you have to perform all five to get the best results. But you can still obtain some relief if you do less if the pain gets to be too much. Let the pain be your guide. Since this is my story, I want to relate to you that I just happen to like to begin my exercises with the TO AND FRO after I assume the proper upside-down position. I hook one of my thumbs near the angle of my jaw and do the same with my other thumb. Then I spread the rest of my fingers on opposing sides of my face over and behind my ears in comfortable positions.

I bend my body forward at the waist and do abdominal crunches. I raise my head, neck, and torso as high and as forward as I can. Sometimes, I hold this position for a second or two and then go back to neutral position. From there, I move my body backward as far as it would go, then go back to neutral position to complete the set. I usually do ten repetitions. Then I proceed to do the next set of exercises after a couple of seconds' rest. I believe a second or two of rest in between sets of exercises was good for my body. Of course, you can do away with this rest period if you are pressed for time. If my low back pain permits me to do only two exercises, the TWISTER will be my second choice.

Exercise II

THE TWISTER

Starting from the usual neutral position, I twist my whole body toward the left side at the waist as much turn as my body would allow, then go back to the neutral position.

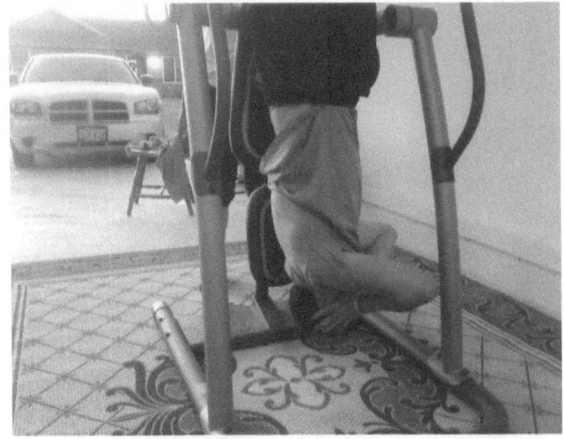

I repeat the process, twisting toward the right and do ten reps.

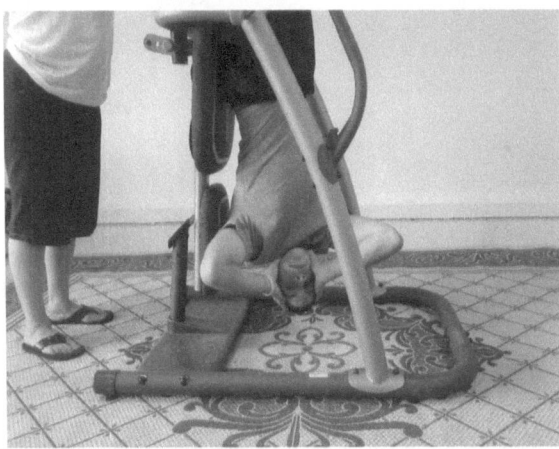

You can definitely do the reverse if you want to, twisting toward the right first to achieve the same results. I firmly believe that among all the exercises I describe here, this is the one exercise that is most efficacious in treating my common low back pain. If I can only do one exercise because of severe acute common low back pain, I will chose to do this one. Completing ten or fewer reps will allow for pain relief

Exercise III

THE SIDE TO SIDE

I start this set the usual way: with my head in the relaxed upside-down position with my thumbs hooked near the angle of my jaw on opposing sides of my face. I flex my body at the waist toward the left as much as I can. Sometimes, I hold the position for a second or two and then go back to the neutral head-down position. Then I repeat the process, bending at the waist toward the right side. Then on to the next set after doing ten reps. You can do this set of exercise even if you can hang only partially upside down (less than ninety degrees) and still reap some common low back pain relief after a longer period of time.

Exercise IV

THE LEFT REVOLUTION

As the name implies, in this set, I swing my torso at the waist around in a wide circle making a complete counterclockwise revolution. I do ten complete counterclockwise revolutions, then return to the neutral head-down position. This is much harder to do with more recent gravity inversion machines because of space limitations while hanging upside down, but I try to do it anyway. The same goes for the next exercise. This exercise could be done very well and with a lot of exaggeration using the Roman chair.

Exercise V

THE RIGHT REVOLUTION

Starting with my head in neutral head-down position, I do this fifth and last set by reversing the direction of the previous set to clockwise rotation. I do ten continuous revolutions before going back to neutral head-down position. After this last set, I slowly but progressively return to the upright position most preferably with someone's help. Most times, I can get up by myself without anyone's help. Like the previous exercise, this exercise can be done extremely well using the Roman chair.

Chapter 6

THE ALTERNATIVES

For individuals who cannot afford to buy a gravity inversion machine, there are other ways to assume the neutral head-down position. I have mentioned earlier the use of chin-up bar and special gravity inversion boots.

Another way is by the use of what is called the Roman chair.

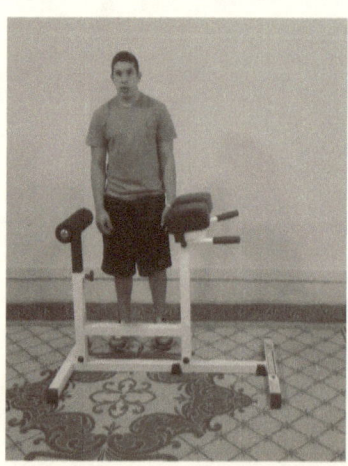

This equipment allowed me in six seconds to assume the head-down neutral position by bending at the waist.

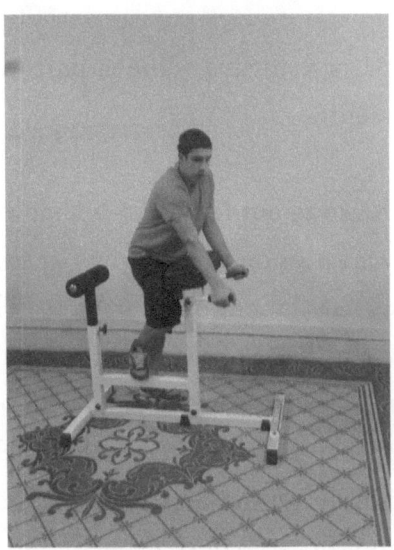

I bought the equipment years ago in Las Vegas, Nevada. My weight is supported at my waist by foam pads. My legs are kept in horizontal position by a horizontal bar at my lower legs, close to my ankles.

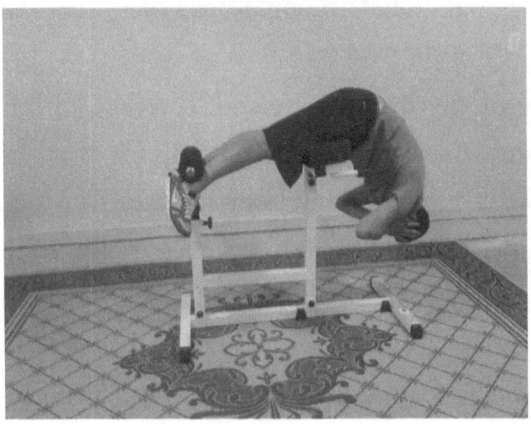

I found out the hard way that it was impossible for me to get on this machine while suffering an attack of acute severe common low back pain. Therefore, I do not recommend the use of the Roman chair for acute severe common low back pain. I use this machine as part of my exercise routine and when I have minor to moderate low back or neck pain relapse, but not for acute severe common low back or neck pain. I always achieve pain relief after I do my exercises on this machine.

I imagine you can use an outdoor chin-up bar to hang upside down. You have to hook your knees on the chin-up bar to do so. You can then proceed to do the exercises I mentioned previously. I must say that your back and/or neck pain must be of the minor to moderate variety. If you have severe common low back or neck pain, I believe it is impossible for you to get into the proper position even with somebody else's help. Of course, I have not tried using this alternative because I have the gravity inversion machine and the Roman chair.

I have already mentioned the use of chin-up bar in between doorjambs. I used this method at the very beginning of my quest to achieve low back pain relief, of which I was very successful.

Lastly, one of my friends, Nelson Torres, LVN, did not have a gravity inversion machine. Unfortunately for him, he developed a progressively worsening common low back pain. By a lucky coincidence, he owned an upright triceps extension exercise machine he bought on sale at Walmart. Instead of using the machine to exercise the triceps muscle, I suggested to him to turn around and hang by his elbows with his back against the foam backing and let both legs hang down freely. From that position, I encouraged him to do my five complete sets of gravity traction exercises. I could not call it gravity inversion at that time because he was hanging right side up. He did his exercises daily as I had suggested. Several days passed without any relief of his common low back pain. When he did not get any low back pain relief after two weeks, he said he was getting discouraged. Because he believed he had nothing to lose and he did not want surgery, he continued on with his upright gravity traction exercises even if he lost hope that he will ever experience relief from his common low back pain. After twenty-one days, he reported to me that he woke up one morning with no more common low back pain. He was pain free for over three weeks when he went overseas for vacation. He did not have recurrence of common low back pain the whole month he was on vacation. From that time on, he informed me that he only does the gravity traction exercises when he has minor relapse of his common low back pain. He keeps his gravity traction exercise equipment in his exercise room at his home.

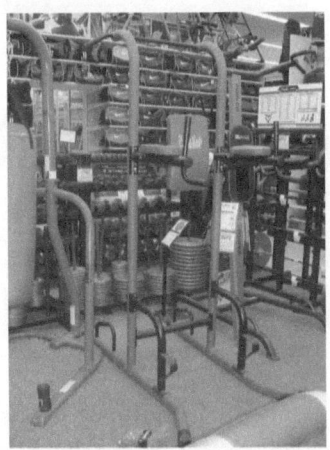

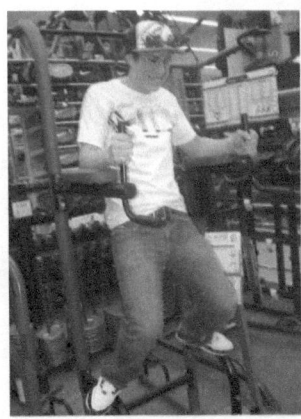 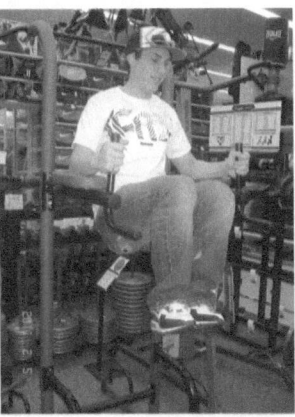

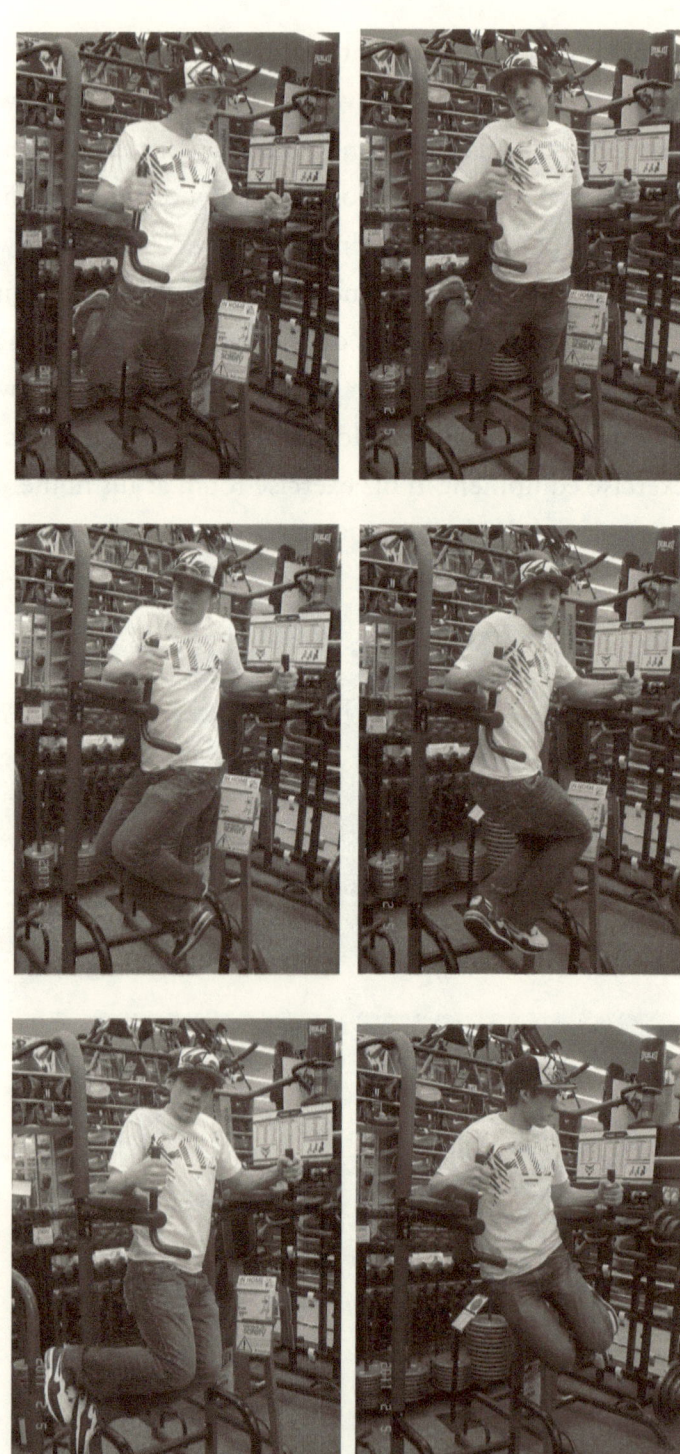

Chapter 7

MY EXPERIENCES

I want you, my faithful reader, to get on with it and achieve your own common low back pain relief, then in your spare time, read on about what I went through all these years. I have been doing gravity traction (inversion) with exercises for slightly over twenty years. I have experienced and learned a lot. All the while, I was always successful in getting rid of my common low back pain and minor neck pain. It is storytelling time. It is my hope that you will learn from and might be entertained by my experiences. I learned by trial and error. I had several recurrences of my minor common low back and neck pain. I lost count. I achieved complete relief by using my method every time pain recurred.

For example, I was invited to Nelson's son's birthday party held at his residence. A few days prior, I started having minor twinges of back pain. I ignored the pain. During a tour of his house, I noticed immediately his gravity traction exercise machine. I asked his permission to use this equipment. After doing my complete set of gravity traction exercises, I was pain free. Subsequently, I was able to enjoy myself fully for the remainder of the party.

I had a couple of severe acute low back pain episodes. I am sad to report that recurrences are common with common low back or neck pain. My back is so unforgiving that by bending at the waist while lifting a heavy object always gives me recurrence of my low back pain. But the good news is that by using my method, I always achieve common low back or neck pain relief after ninety seconds of exercises for minor to moderate common low back pain or seventy-two hours for acute severe common low back pain.

I experienced severe acute low back pain one Saturday morning in the summer of 2008. I went to an auction that day. I remembered what happened that day very clearly. I won at the auction a kerosene can full of metal pegboard hangers. I picked up this heavy can by bending at my waist. I carried the can to a chair without any pain. I sat down and rested for a couple of minutes. When I got up, a very sharp, shooting pain pierced my back. Any minor movement produced excruciating pain. I thought that what I felt must be what my patients, who underwent emergency spine surgery, experienced. People who witnessed my suffering asked if I was having a heart attack. I said no. I wanted to lie down, but I can't because I was still at the auction. Any small muscle movement, even coughing, brought immediate severe pain and back muscle spasm. Even stepping one foot at a time to walk was very painful. I wondered how I was going to get home. As a last resort, I called my friend, Sergio Andrade, to help me load the articles I won at the auction onto my truck. I managed with great difficulty to drive my truck back to my house. Sergio helped me unload my truck when we got to our destination. After I thanked Sergio profusely, I laid down to rest. That was all I wanted to do. And that was all I could do. The main reason was that as long as I lay down flat on my back and did not move a muscle, I did not have pain. The instant I moved a muscle, severe shooting low back pain and muscles spasms ensued. I was tempted to go to the Emergency Room at Shannon Hospital. I knew if I did that I could end up having emergency back surgery. I could not afford to be sidelined by surgery. No work, no pay. I needed the money. To earn the money, I had to be back at work Monday—two days away. I felt confident that my method combining gravity traction with exercises would get me out of my predicament. I was eventually proven correct.

That same afternoon, two things were immediately evident to me. One, I tried to get on the Roman chair, but could not because of excruciating pain. Two, the only way I could get on the gravity inversion machine was with the help of my wife, presently my ex. I needed help to secure my feet into the special boots. I definitely could not do it by myself. It was impossible because of severe pain and muscle spasms. I needed help to get on and off the machine and to get into upside-down position. The pain would only allow me to do two repetitions of each set of five exercises. That was it. Then I lay flat in bed and slept. My helper asked me if I wanted to take pain medications. I said no. I did not have pain as long as I did not move. I slept the rest of the day and night.

I woke up early the following day, Sunday, feeling slightly better. The pain was much less. I could move around with less pain. I dared not move a lot for fear of making the pain worse. I was able to walk to the kitchen to eat breakfast. Around 10:00 a.m., I felt adventurous enough to get on the gravity inversion machine without any help. I put on the boots, got on the machine, and hung upside down without any problem. I performed my complete set of five exercises with ten repetitions each without difficulty. I took it easy the rest of the day. I watched TV, but slept mostly. After I woke up from each sleep period, I felt much better. By evening Sunday, I was more mobile. I felt like I could go to work the following day, which I did.

At 5:30 a.m. Monday morning, my low back pain was gone. I woke up refreshed. I twisted, turned, and got up from bed without any problem. I went to work without anybody knowing about my severe acute low back pain episode two days earlier. I mentioned it to some of my coworkers, but nobody seemed alarmed or interested with what I just went through. It seemed to them so unbelievable that I went from having acute severe low back pain to no back pain in seventy-two hours. That afternoon, I was able to do several repetitions of jumping jacks exercise. For me, I was just thankful that I was able to get back to work after the weekend was over.

Chapter 8

THE EVER AFTER

Recurrences—whether mild, moderate, or severe—are common occurrence with common low back and/or neck pain. With regards to recurrences of minor low back pain and/or neck pain, especially at the end of a day's work and being on my feet for several hours, I just get on my gravity inversion machine, do my exercises, and get off the machine. Once upright, my low back and/or neck pain was always gone, replaced by a hollow feeling in my back and/or neck. Then, I take it easy for the rest of the day and wait for the next episode of recurrence of low back and/or neck pain. The pain-free intervals can last from weeks to months. I never had trouble with insomnia because of common low back and/or neck pain.

As I have mentioned earlier, I treated my common low back pain as close to its onset as possible. It took me several days of ninety second per day gravity inversion exercises to achieve complete relief at the outset. But I achieved my goal eventually. I am happy to report that along the way I became aware that minor neck pain was also relieved by my method. I was never unlucky enough to have acute severe neck pain, like from whiplash injury. I firmly believe that the best way to treat common low back pain and/or neck pain is to treat it as close to its onset as possible, no matter how minor the pain maybe and no matter how young or old the individual may be. Early onset herniated disc responds well to my method. Severe slipped (herniated) disc or sliding herniated disk may not respond well to my method especially if the herniation has been around for a very long time. After a long period of time, vertebral bone spurs develop. Once you have vertebral body bone spurs, it is perhaps too late to do gravity inversion with exercises. I am afraid that the bone spurs will somehow break off and cut the spinal cord or nerve branches during the exercises. I could be wrong. But I would rather err on the conservative side. If you want to give my method a try anyways, despite you having vertebral bone spurs, you do it at your own risk. Let the pain be your guide. Do less vigorous exercises and less repetitions. I subscribe to the notion that "no venture, no gain."

I cannot say with a lot of conviction that my method will work for individuals who have had spine surgery because I did not have spine surgery. I would not recommend my method to these individuals. The same thing goes for individuals who have unhealed vertebral (spine) fractures. Once the fractures heal, then maybe. I must say that I feel very lucky and blessed to have discovered my method of relieving common low back and/or neck pain when I needed it the most while in my thirties. Even if I do not have low back pain, I sometimes perform my method as part of my exercise regimen. I believe that gravity inversion exercises will promote healthier and stronger backs, make recurrences less likely, and if one does have recurrence, the pain, no matter how severe, can be treated successfully within seventy-two hours' time. Quite possibly, one can also gain one inch in height with being upside down for prolonged periods of time. Another good thing is that your initial investment of gravity inversion equipment is not wasted, not by a long shot. I am sure that everyone one of us has one or two family members or close friends who will eventually develop common low back and/or neck pain. This equipment can then be handed down to those who need it the most. Or you can sell the equipment to another low back pain or neck pain victim. Isn't it wonderful?

As a parting thought, now that you know what I have known for years about my method of successfully treating common low back and/or neck pain, the question you should ask yourself is not whether my method will work for you because I am sure it will. But rather, the question you should ask yourself is this: are you motivated and brave enough to get into the proper position and do the exercises? I wish you the best.

Chapter 9

(AND MORE)

I will describe to you other off-label uses of certain stuffs that worked for me and for others outside of common low back or neck pain arena. You don't have to believe in what I say here, and you don't have to follow what I did. If, however, you are a bit curious, I invite you to try, but do them entirely at your own risk. So after being warned, let us begin.

1. Heat, the noble solution

The hair dryer is one common household appliance that has many off-label uses. I have used a hair dryer to treat and cure minor skin infections from minor cuts, scratches, abrasions, and solitary pimples with good success. My recent onset inflamed hemorrhoids were also treated with great effectiveness. I believe the heat from the hair dryer kills the bacteria at the site of infection. I have treated jellyfish stings successfully. I believe that the heat from the dryer denatures the protein in the poison, and the body's immune system clears away the debris. I was fortunate enough not to be exposed to poison ivy, so I do not know if the heat from the hair dryer will cure poison ivy exposure. If I were exposed, I will definitely try this form of heat treatment after washing thoroughly the affected area. I also treated minor skin itching from many causes with heat. If the skin itching was due to dry skin, I followed the heat treatment with baby oil or body lotion to prolong the itching relief. The common denominator for the hair dryer being so effective is the intense heat it produces. I call it cooking the germs in minor skin infections, and cooking the poison in jellyfish stings or skin itching. I apply heat from the hair dryer until I could not tolerate the pain any longer. Then I point the hair dryer away from the treated area until the pain subsides. I repeat the process three or four more times. Then I quit for the day and leave the treated area alone for at least twenty-four hours. I may or may not repeat the process the following day. Sometimes, I repeat the process for three or more successive days. The skin itching is usually replaced with pain. When the pain goes away, the itching is also gone. For minor skin infections, pain at the site of infection is already present. This pain should not deter you from proceeding with the heat treatment. The redness of the skin infection is usually gone in seventy-two hours after a few seconds of heat treatment per day. I do not recommend this form of heat therapy to persons who had lost their heat sensation to the treated area, like those who suffer from diabetic peripheral neuropathy, stroke, or physical trauma. If, however, you have a friend, relative, or trusted person apply the heat, that person must place one of their fingers in the blow dryer heat stream while applying the heat to the victim's affected area and use their own pain to determine how much heat to apply. I believe this will prevent the treated area from being burned. I cannot stress strongly enough that you do this at your own risk.

Another cheap, readily available, portable, high heat source I know of is the electric handheld paint stripper. The idea behind this particular paint stripper is that it uses extremely high heat to peel off paint from wood or metal, and the supplied scraper is used to scrape off the paint into a disposal container.

I want to mention a couple of infestations that may respond well to high heat treatment by a paint stripper mentioned above. One is caused by a member of the animal kingdom. The offending organism is the lowly bedbug. If you have not seen the TV documentary about bedbug infestation, I'm here to pass on to you the fact that bedbugs die if they are subjected to temperatures above 120 degrees Fahrenheit for at least thirty minutes. If, however, you apply high heat from a paint stripper, you will "cook" the live bedbugs and their eggs in less than a minute.

Another infestation worthy of mention is house infestation with a member of the plant kingdom, the black mold. A house infested with the black mold is a house condemned, a total loss. Evidently, several chemicals have been tried to kill the black mold without much success. Black mold is a fungus. It is alive. A mushroom is a fungus. Have you ever tried eating cooked mushrooms at home or in a restaurant? Tastes good, doesn't it? The mushroom dies when cooked, and you are treated to a delicious meal. You can also kill or cook black mold with high heat; however, please don't eat it. Heat is just one effective and inexpensive way to get rid of black mold. *Use caution* when using high heat around your house. You can start a fire unintentionally. Take steps not to burn your house. Have water readily available and spray cold water to treated areas so treated areas will not ignite spontaneously. Finally, it is best to treat both infestations as soon as possible.

2. Glue me down

If you are a do-it-yourself person like me, you probably have tried numerous brands of glue, with varying degrees of success. The most effective type of glue I have accidentally found is not marketed as glue at all. The stuff is marketed as a *rifle bedding compound*. The fortuitous accident happened to me this way. I am an avid hunter and relentlessly pursued anything that improved the accuracy of my rifles. I applied this bedding compound to the wooden stock of one of my rifles. Serendipitously, I forgot to apply the release agent unto the barrel of the rifle. I reassembled the rifle. Twenty-four hours later, I found out to my dismay that I could not remove the barrel from the rifle stock no matter how hard I tried. Then it hit me. If I wanted to join two similar or dissimilar materials together without it coming apart ever, I could use this bedding compound like glue. To date, I have used this bedding compound to join just about any two broken or intact pieces of furniture, wood, china, plastics, and metals with great success. I even used this compound to make new handles for kitchen utensils with excellent results. The mentioned bedding compound is sold at Field and Stream, Texas Gun Shop, and Outdoorsman here in San Angelo, Texas. It is called ACRAGLAS. It comes in two different packagings. The *green package* contains a jelly-type resin and hardener. I used this type to join broken pieces with large gaps between them. I also used it to make handles for knives and other kitchen utensils. The *red package* contains a resin and hardener of syrupy consistency. I used this type of bedding compound to join together pieces with minimal gaps between them like fine china, glass, or plastic. Follow the mixing instructions. Use ACRAGLAS with caution because the vapor it gives off is toxic. Make sure you mix the resin and hardener in a well-ventilated area. One disadvantage of ACRAGLAS over regularly marketed glues in the open market is that it takes twenty-four hours for the bedding compound to get very hard. I usually use tape to hold the pieces together that I want joined and let the bedding compound harden for twenty-four hours. I have used clamps to hold pieces to be joined together for twenty-four hours. I have tried to make the glue harden faster using heat with no success. I have tried using more hardener than recommended, but it still took over four hours for the glue to harden. I do not know if hastening the hardening process makes the joint brittle. Remember: use the releasing agent if there are pieces you do not want glued together because once the glue sets, you cannot take the pieces apart without wrecking your work of art.

Warning: You cannot glue together successfully two hard objects with ACRAGLAS if either has a very smooth surface. The two objects will come apart after the glue hardens. The main reason is that the glue does not have a surface to hang on to. You must provide this rough surface. I have used coarse sandpaper with good success. I am most successful if I use the sharp point of a blade to make crisscross pattern on the surfaces I want joined. I made sure the glue gets into the microscopic crevices that the blade has made. After twenty-four hours, I could not separate the two joined objects.

3. Fish story

This story actually involves real fish, more accurately, how to attract fish so you can enjoy swimming with fish while snorkeling or scuba diving. This is for vacationers who go snorkeling and/or scuba diving. Most often, when one goes snorkeling or scuba diving all one can see are these almost microscopic fish swimming around. Bigger fish are nowhere to be found unless you are in a place like Hanauma Bay on the island of Oahu in Hawaii. I discovered a surefire trick to attract fish inexpensively. I first tried this trick successfully while we were on vacation in Mexico. I took bread and assorted pastries from the morning buffet line during breakfast. Hid my goodies inside a plastic bag and placed my bounty inside my pants pocket. I leisurely went snorkeling. I saw only one to two small fish swimming around. I took out the goodies inside my pants pocket. I opened the plastic container underwater and began to spread all around me small pieces of bread and pastries. Almost instantly, as if on cue, I was surrounded by fish of varying colors and sizes. The fish were all around me until I ran out of goodies. Then they swam away and disappeared. I repeated this trick several times in different locations with the same degree of success.

4. The movement

And finally, I would like to mention a very touchy subject for most people. I have only thirty minutes to get ready for work Monday to Friday. To accomplish this, I have to dispose of my bodily waste quickly before taking a shower. I use exercises with dumbbells while sitting on the commode to make me have bowel movement expeditiously. It takes just a couple of minutes, sometimes less, to get me going. I use exercise, using two five-pound and one forty-pound dumbbells, as a fast-acting laxative. I use two five-pound dumbbells for my warm-up, one in each hand. I hold both five-pound dumbbells at chest level. I execute alternating dumbbell forward strikes up to fifty repetitions. You can do more if it pleases you. I follow my warm-up exercise with the main exercise sets using the forty-pound dumbbell. I begin by placing the forty-pound dumbbell to my right side and placing my left hand on my thigh nearest my left knee for body support. I lift the dumbbell straight up with my right hand as high as I can on my right side. I believe this exercise is called lateral dumbbell raises. I perform ten repetitions. I repeat the process on my left side using my left hand to complete the first set of exercises. Then I place the forty-pound weight on the floor in front of me. I use my right hand to do dumbbell biceps curls with ten repetitions. I repeat the process using my left hand and do ten repetitions. This completes the second set of exercises. My last exercise consists of lifting the forty-pound dumbbell using both hands straight up over my head, then slowly letting the dumbbell drop behind me This part is called the dumbbell triceps curl. Slowly, I bring the dumbbell back to the starting position. I do five repetitions with this exercise. You are welcome to do more reps if you so desire. At the conclusion of these exercises, I am done doing number 2. Then, I hit the shower.

Worthwhile and significant side effects of these set of exercises are that they act as potent stimulant and antidepressant. I wake up faster than drinking a cup of coffee or any other stimulant. I feel so refreshed that after my early morning exercises, I feel ready to tackle whatever I may come across that day. I feel good and wide awake. Sometimes I feel depressed that I have to get up so early in the morning that I have to drag myself out of bed. After exercising, my depression is history.

The absence of *depression, common low back pain and/or neck pain, worries, insomnia* makes my life worth living—full of happiness, peace, gratitude, and wonder.

Index